The Mouse's House

Baby Shiatsu
Gentle Touch to Help your Baby Thrive
Karin Kalbantner-Wernicke and Tina Haase
Foreword by Dr. Steffen Fischer
Illustrated by Monika Werneke
ISBN 978 1 84819 104 4
eISBN 978 0 85701 086 5

Ladybird's Remarkable Relaxation
How children (and frogs, dogs, flamingos and dragons) can use yoga relaxation
to help deal with stress, grief, bullying and lack of confidence
Michael Chissick
Illustrated by Sarah Peacock
ISBN 978 1 84819 146 4
eISBN 978 0 85701 112 1

Frog's Breathtaking Speech
How Children (and Frogs) Can Use Yoga Breathing to
Deal with Anxiety, Anger and Tension
Michael Chissick
Illustrated by Sarah Peacock
ISBN 978 1 84819 091 7
eISBN 978 0 85701 074 2

Principles of Reflexology
What it is, how it works, and what it can do for you
Nicola Hall
Part of the Discovering Holistic Health series
ISBN 978 1 84819 137 2
eISBN 978 0 85701 108 4

The Mouse's House

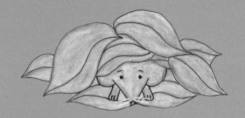

CHILDREN'S REFLEXOLOGY FOR BEDTIME OR ANYTIME

SUSAN QUAYLE
ILLUSTRATED BY MELISSA MULDOON
FOREWORD BY BARBARA SCOTT

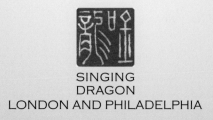

SINGING
DRAGON
LONDON AND PHILADELPHIA

This edition published in 2015
by Singing Dragon
an imprint of Jessica Kingsley Publishers
73 Collier Street
London N1 9BE, UK
and
400 Market Street, Suite 400
Philadelphia, PA 19106, USA

www.singingdragon.com

First edition published by Create Space in 2013

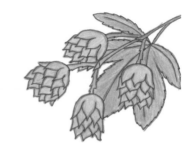

Library of Congress Cataloging in Publication Data
A CIP catalog record for this book is available from the Library of Congress

British Library Cataloguing in Publication Data
A CIP catalogue record for this book is available from the British Library

ISBN 978 1 84819 247 8
eISBN 978 0 85701 193 0

Printed and bound in China

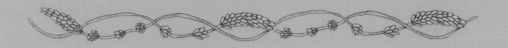

For Ariadne and Cassius and all the children I have met through their mothers' feet.
SQ

For Luis and Ewan.
MM

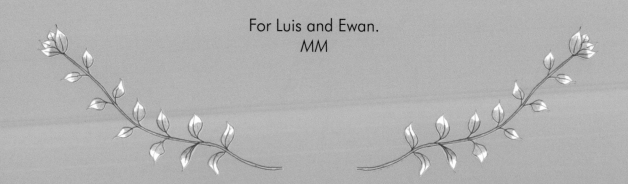

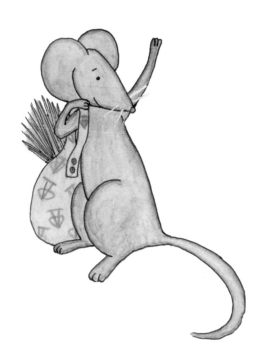

Contents

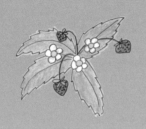

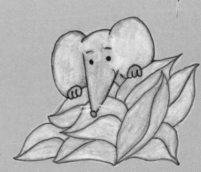

Foreword

Over my many years in practice I have worked with a great number of parents, babies and children and have seen how valuable a tool reflexology can be. There have been numerous occasions when I have shown a distressed mother how to work reflex points that will help not only to calm a fractious baby, but also to improve health and well-being.

It was with great joy that I read this delightful book. It encapsulates those reflex points that are of most benefit to young children in the most beautifully creative way.

Enabling a parent and child to engage with each other in such a healing way for both of them can only be a positive thing.

I am sure that those parents and children who are fortunate enough to experience this book will derive enormous pleasure and benefit from it.

Good health and many blessings to you all, Big and Small.

Barbara Scott

Chair, Association of Reproductive Reflexologists

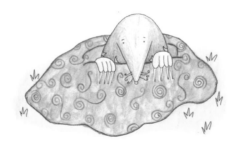

Introduction

This children's reflexology programme has been designed to enable parents, carers, family and friends to offer children the benefits of reflexology in a way that is fun, relaxing and supports natural bonding.

Reflexology is a gentle, non-invasive complementary therapy that can help with many common ailments of childhood. The feet contain reflex points that correspond to different parts of the body. When these reflexes are manipulated it helps to ease problems within that area of the body as well as to support the body's own ability to self-heal. As a reflexologist I have worked with many babies, toddlers and children, as well as adults, and have seen how effective it can be.

As well as offering invaluable therapeutic benefits, this book is designed to aid in the bonding process between the adult and the child. Reading this story at bedtime and performing the actions on the child's foot will create a sense of quality time, fun and positive touch between you. The time you spend relating these stories in a positive way will offer help, distraction, comfort and a feeling of safety at other times in your child's life. In my experience children can be brought back from utter distress with a comforting distraction that is familiar to them.

It is also a way for parents and carers to offer help at times when they feel helpless. A child suffering pain from a condition such as constipation, colic or teething is heart-breaking for a parent who feels unable to offer any relief. With these stories there is the opportunity not only to help comfort them but to actually relieve their discomfort.

Repeated regularly these stories can help to support your child's good health. They can also offer you the chance to catch a problem before it develops and becomes out of control. Regular treatment can relieve conditions such as constipation, colic and teething before they become a problem. Reflexology can also be used alongside conventional medicine to support

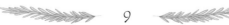

more serious conditions such as asthma and epilepsy. As a complementary therapist I would never encourage anyone to stop taking prescribed medication unless it had been sanctioned by their doctor.

The Gentle Touch

When working on very young children – newborns, babies and toddlers – it is essential that you use a very light touch. Their young feet are very sensitive. Their bones and musculature will be undeveloped and their reflexes will be very sensitive. It is unlikely that you will hurt your child, unless you use a very strong pressure, but it will not be conducive to the relaxing and positive results we are after. Never perform reflexology on a child when you are feeling angry as it is important that the experience remains a positive one for everyone, especially them.

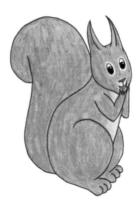

Basic Reflexology Techniques

Caterpillar

The caterpillar, or thumb and finger walking, will be the most used technique. The illustration shows thumb walking. Slide the tip of the thumb forward by extending the first joint as shown, then raise the joint to the original position by rolling the tip of the thumb in place, and repeat. The tip will move slowly forward in very small steps like a caterpillar walking. Finger walking is very similar but uses the index finger instead of the thumb.

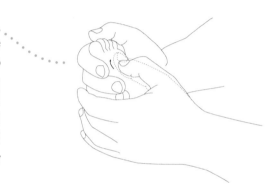

Butterfly

This is done using the outside edge of both thumbs to gently stroke the reflex, pulling away from each other. Useful when working the Lung reflex. Hold the foot as shown in the image and stroke the reflex gently by moving the thumbs apart. Lift the thumbs and return them to the original position to repeat.

Finger Stroking

This is basically what it says. Use a gentle motion with a light pressure, stroking the foot downwards with the fingers.

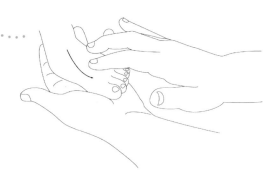

Hand Stroking

Gently glide your hands, palms down, over the feet, completely enveloping them with their warmth and comfort. Glide up the foot toward the leg and then down the sides before starting over. Very relaxing and a lovely way to begin and end the story.

Kissing

This is your baby, grandchild or little person that you care for. Add a nurturing dimension with kissing and playing and silliness. Bring love and play into the story. Use puppets, toys and funny voices. There are no rules – do what you need to do to make it work for you and your child. To begin with just get them used to having their feet touched throughout the story. There is no hurry, you have their whole childhood ahead of you. Whatever happens is OK, as long as your intention is positive.

The Story and How to Use this Book

This story is based around a group of animal characters. The intention is that each animal represents a particular reflex area. The central character in this book is Mouse. She represents the Solar Plexus, which is very important in all conditions related to pain, discomfort, stress and anxiety. You will return to her reflex regularly to help your child feel calm.

Each written page of the story has a diagram of the feet in the corner showing the reflexes that you should be working, with written instructions on what to do. The story will provide a general reflexology treatment for your child. This means that the main reflexes will be manipulated if you follow the instructions alongside the foot maps on each page. A general treatment is a lovely way to start the day, to end the day before bedtime or to offer as a distraction throughout the day when a child is bored, tired or upset. There are hundreds of ways in which stories can be used to aid children, and this one has another dimension to add to its value. I hope you have fun with it.

If you are using this book with young children, say between one and three years old, you might find it easier to just read it to them as a story at first. This allows the child (and you!) to become familiar with the story and the characters. Children in this age group often find it difficult to sit still and may be resistant to having their feet touched initially. You might like to try just holding their feet while you read the story before progressing on to manipulating the reflexes. Don't give up. If they need the treatment for a condition you can give them the reflexology while they are sleeping until they are ready to receive it while awake. Try not to force them to sit and have the treatment if they are not interested as it may create a barrier to future enjoyment. Some of the young children who have experienced this book were resistant in the beginning but all of them loved it after a very short time.

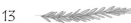

When using the book with babies, including newborns, try to read the story while giving the treatment. Using a sing song voice with a variety of pitches will soothe and calm the baby. In my experience, babies respond positively to warmth and love so make this the intention when reading. Have fun above all else.

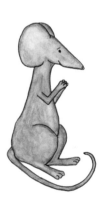

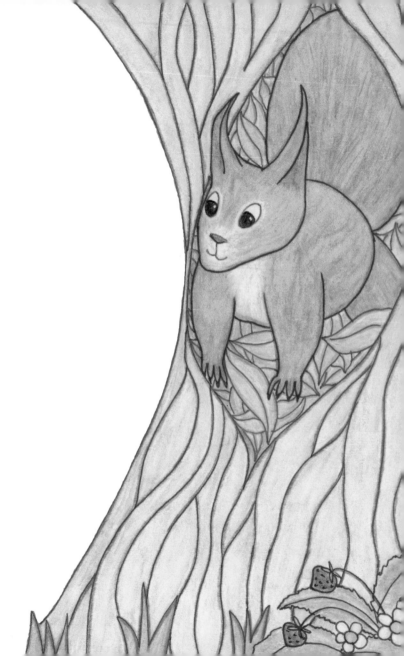

The Reflexes and Characters

The characters in this book each represent a reflex area of the foot. As you visit each of the reflexes, the character representing that reflex appears in the story.

Here are the characters you will meet.

Mouse

Mouse represents the Solar Plexus reflex point. She is the central character and you will return to her again and again.

Squirrel

Squirrel represents the Head, Sinus, Teeth, Eyes and Ear reflexes.

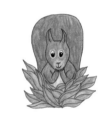

Hare

Hare represents the Lungs and Chest reflexes.

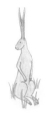

Mole

Mole represents the Digestive System reflexes.

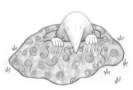

Otter

Otter represents the Lymphatic System reflex.

Snake

Snake represents the Nervous System, Back and Spine reflexes.

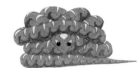

The Mouse's House

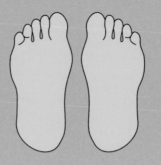

Gently stroke your child's feet to prepare them for their reflexology treatment.

In the ocean blue and deep
Sat an island chain that looked like feet
Joined together with toes of trees
That gently sighed in the salty breeze

On the Island lived a mouse
Who was looking for a cosy house
Where she could sleep the Winter through
And wake up with the Spring anew

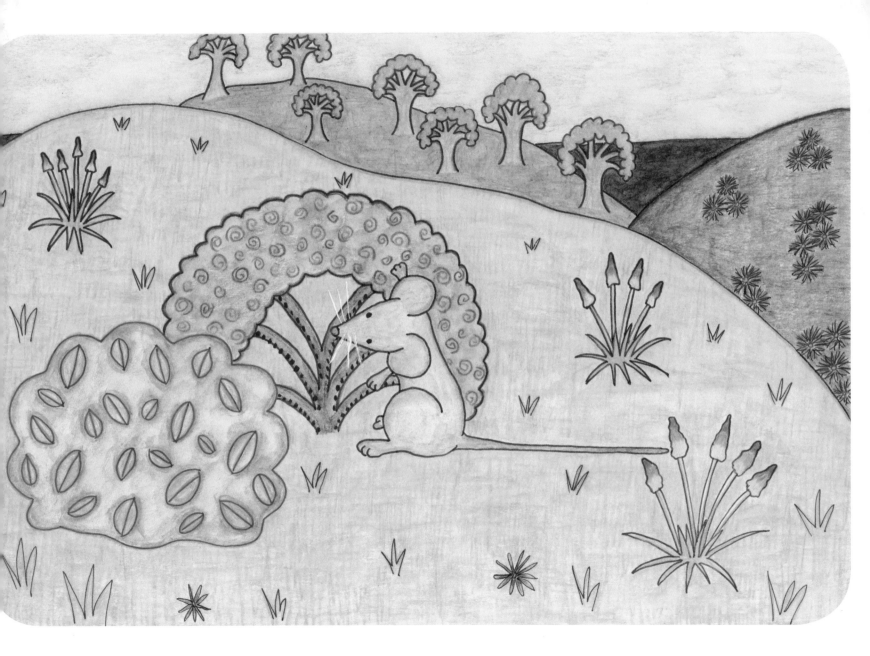

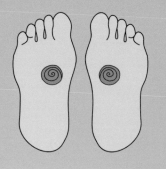

Gently hold with thumbs.

One day she found a little hole
The perfect place to make her home
She snuggled down to go to sleep
But her bed was cold and hard and deep

"I need to make a cosy nest
So I can get a good night's rest
I'll visit all my friends tomorrow
They'll help me make a cosy burrow"

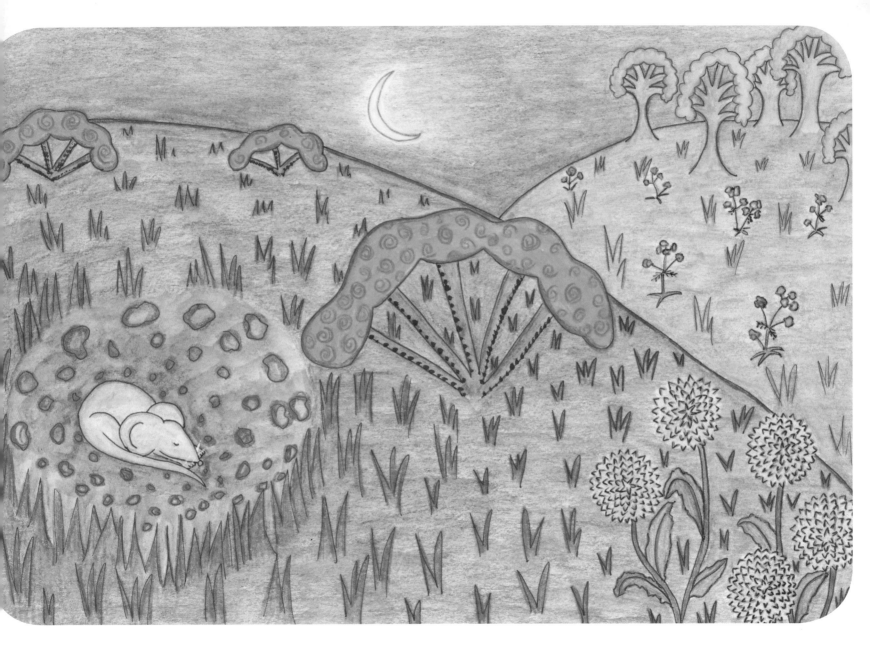

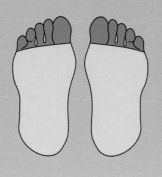

Gently caterpillar
walk up the toes.

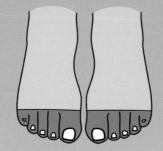

Gently caterpillar walk
down the toes.

Gently circle the
tops of the toes.

In the morning off she set
And Squirrel was the first she met
Squirrel lived amongst the leaves
In a warm, dry hollow of a tree

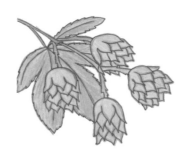

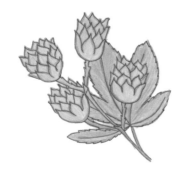

He gave the mouse a sack of leaves
"This is what a new house needs"
"Thank you, Squirrel," said the Mouse
And hurried back to her empty house

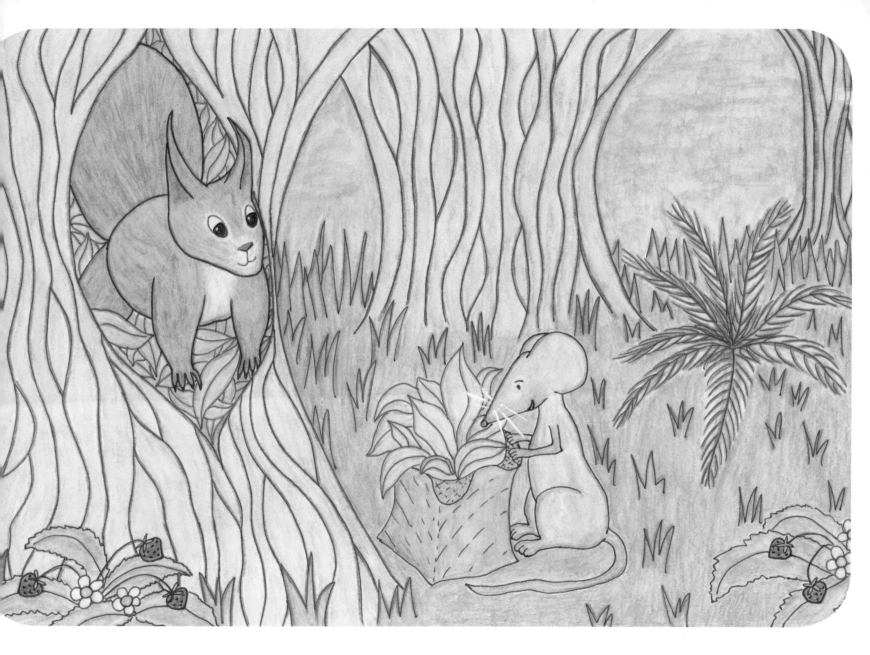

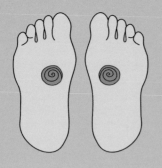

Gently hold with thumbs.

Mouse thought she'd have a little rest
And snuggled down in her leafy nest
Although it wasn't quite as deep
It was cold and hard; Mouse couldn't sleep

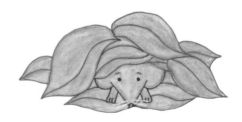

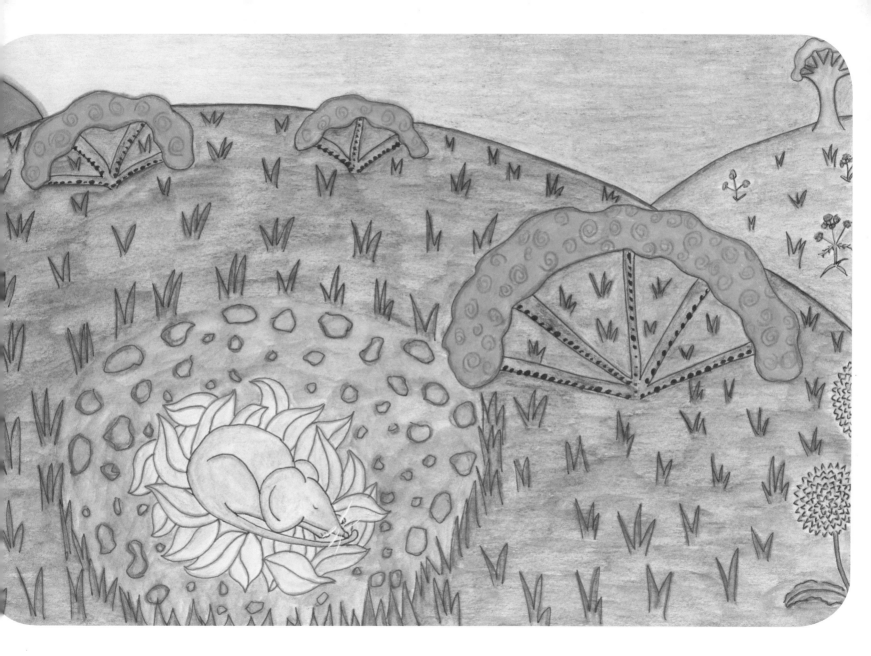

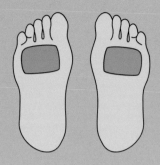

Gently caterpillar walk or butterfly stroke, thumbs together stroking outward.

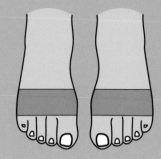

Gently caterpillar walk from the base of the toe down the foot or butterfly stroke, thumbs together stroking outward.

In the morning off she set
And Hare was the first she met
Hare lived high up on the Downs
In a nest beneath the ground

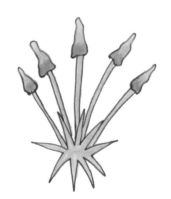

He gave the Mouse a sack of hay
"This makes me want to sleep all day"
"Thank you, Hare," said the Mouse
And hurried back to her chilly house

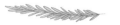

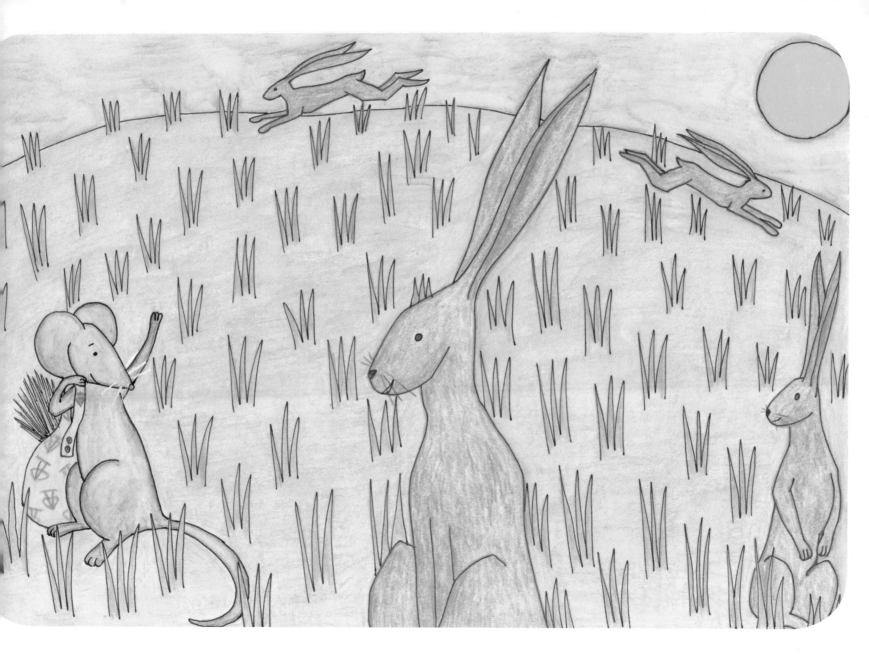

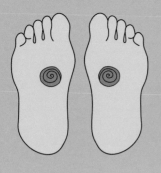

Gently hold with thumbs.

Mouse thought she'd have a little rest
So snuggled down in her crunchy nest
It wasn't quite so hard or deep
But Mouse was cold and couldn't sleep

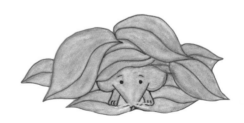

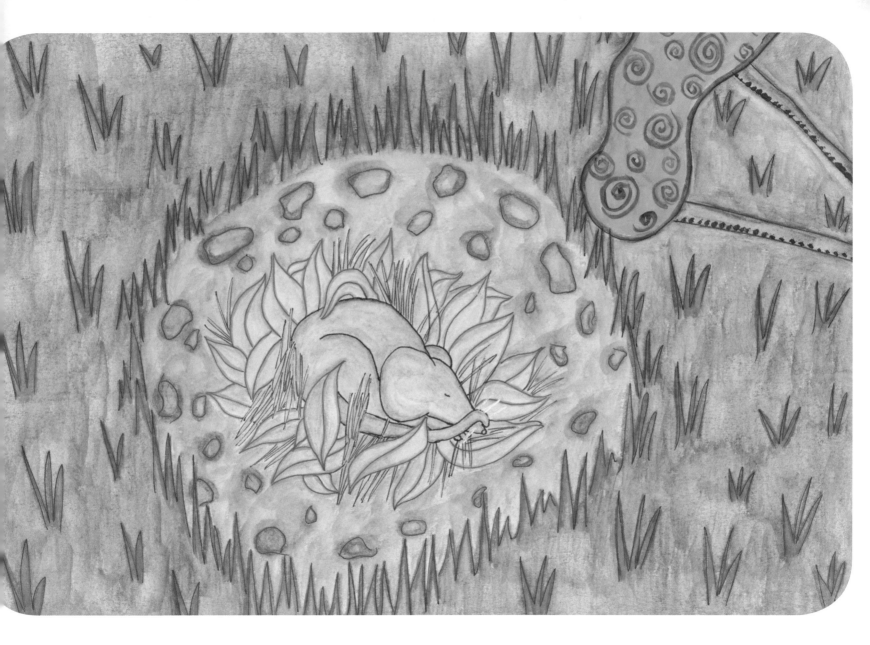

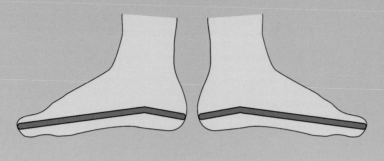

Gently caterpillar walk down the inside of the foot. Slowly work your way back using tiny gentle circular movements.

In the morning off she set
And Snake was the first she met
Curled on a rock beneath the sun
Tasting the air with his tongue

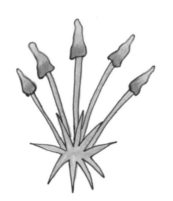

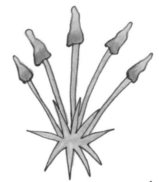

He gave the Mouse a wonderful treat
Herbs and Hops and Lavender sweet
"How lovely, Snake," said the grateful Mouse
And hurried back to her little house

28

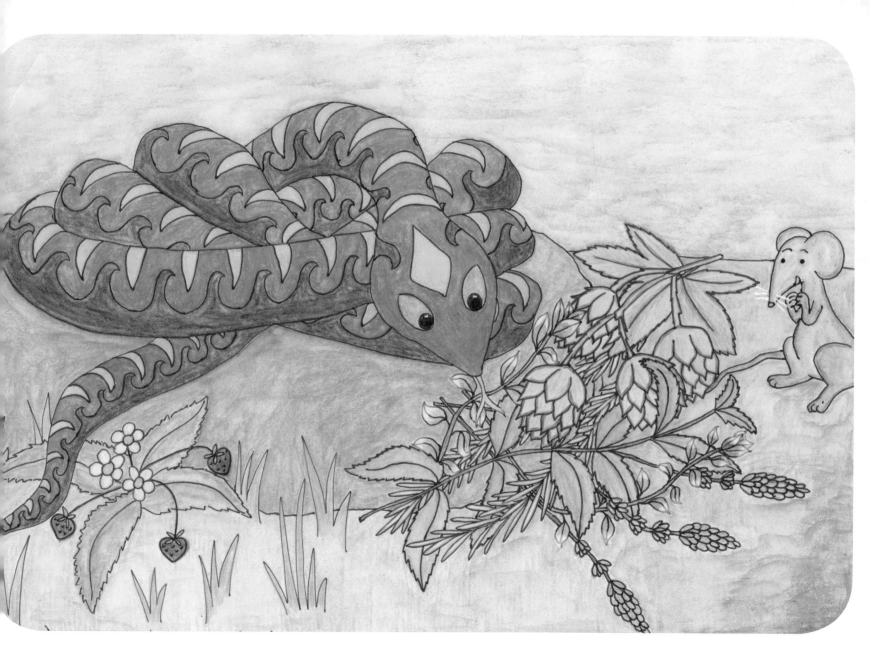

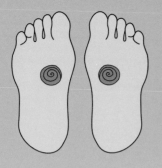

Gently hold with thumbs.

Mouse thought she'd have a little rest
So snuggled down in her posy nest
On fragrant flowers she laid her head
She slept but woke up cold in bed

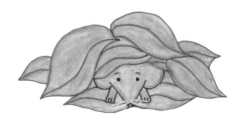

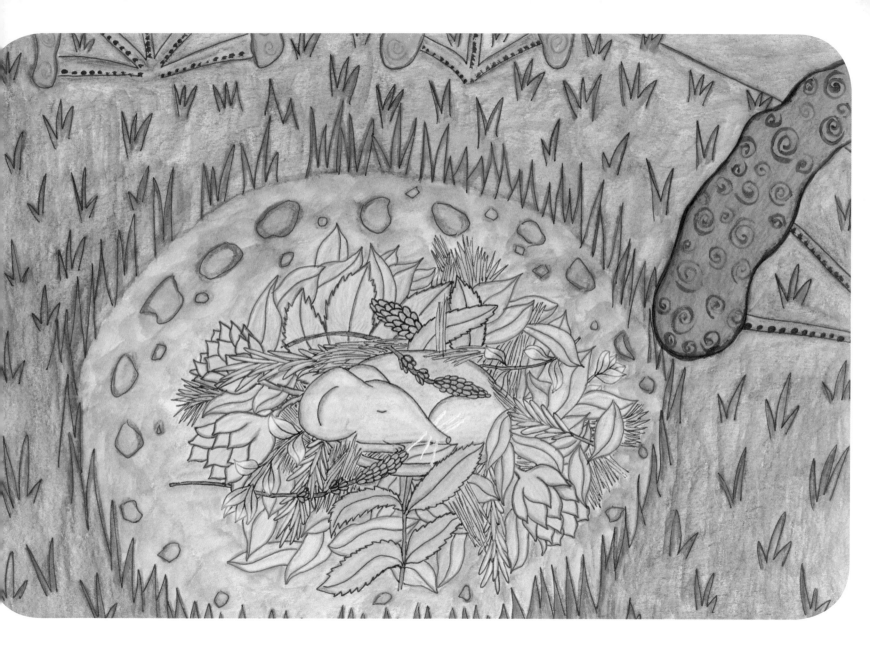

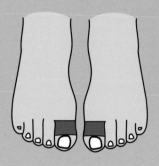

Gently slide your finger down the tops of the big toes.

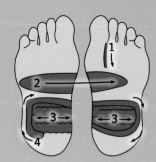

1. Gently slide your thumb down from the join between the big and second toes.
2. Starting on the right foot, slide your thumb across from right to left.
3. Butterfly stroke the lower centre of each foot.
4. Starting on the right foot gently caterpillar walk or use tiny circles to follow the horseshoe.

In the morning off she set
And Mole was the first she met
Mole appeared within a mound
Of soil he'd dug from underground

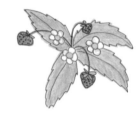

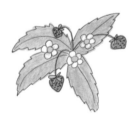

He gave the Mouse a sack all white
Of thistledown, a lovely sight
"Thank you, Mole," said the Mouse
And hurried back to her cosy house

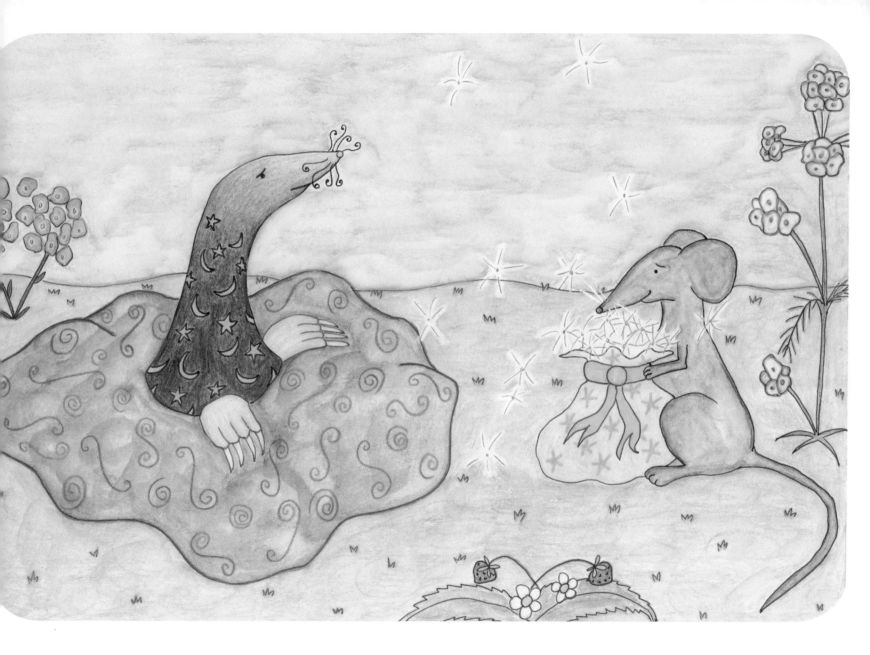

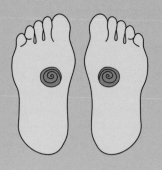

Gently hold with thumbs.

Mouse thought she'd have a little rest
So snuggled down in her cosy nest
It was better than it was before
But she felt it needed something more

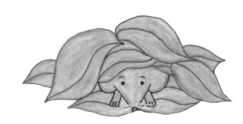

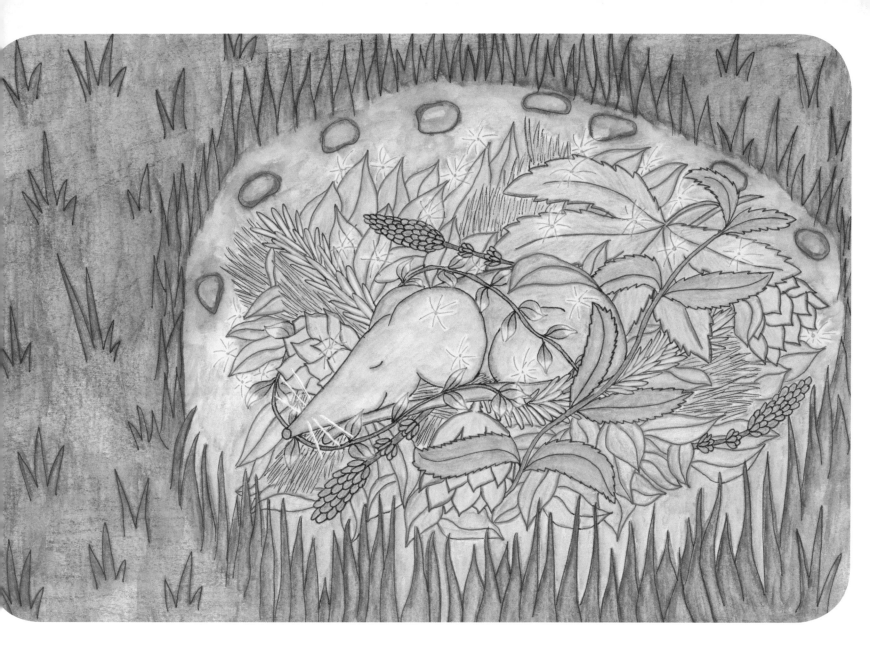

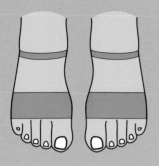

Caterpillar walk from the base of the toes down the top of the foot. Butterfly stroke the top of the foot.

Gently using tiny circles work your way around the top of the ankle, gently stoking up the leg.

In the morning off she set
And Otter was the first she met
He lived above the emerald socks
That, at low tide, adorned the rocks

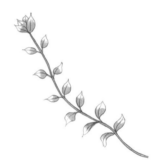

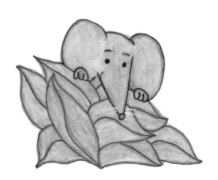

He gave the Mouse a sack of down
"The Eider Duck leaves me a mound"
"Thank you, Otter," said the Mouse
And hurried back to her cosy house

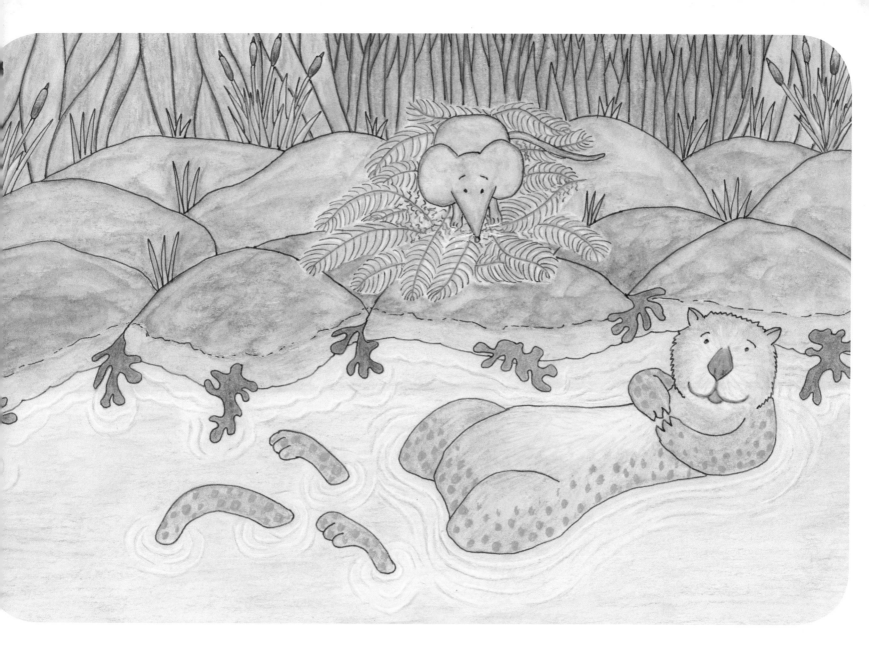

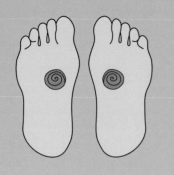

Gently hold with thumbs.

Mouse thought she'd have a little rest
So snuggled down in her cosy nest
Which wasn't cold or hard or deep
Mouse instantly fell fast asleep

All that work had worn her out
That she was tired there was no doubt
She slept right through the winter long
And woke when all the frosts had gone

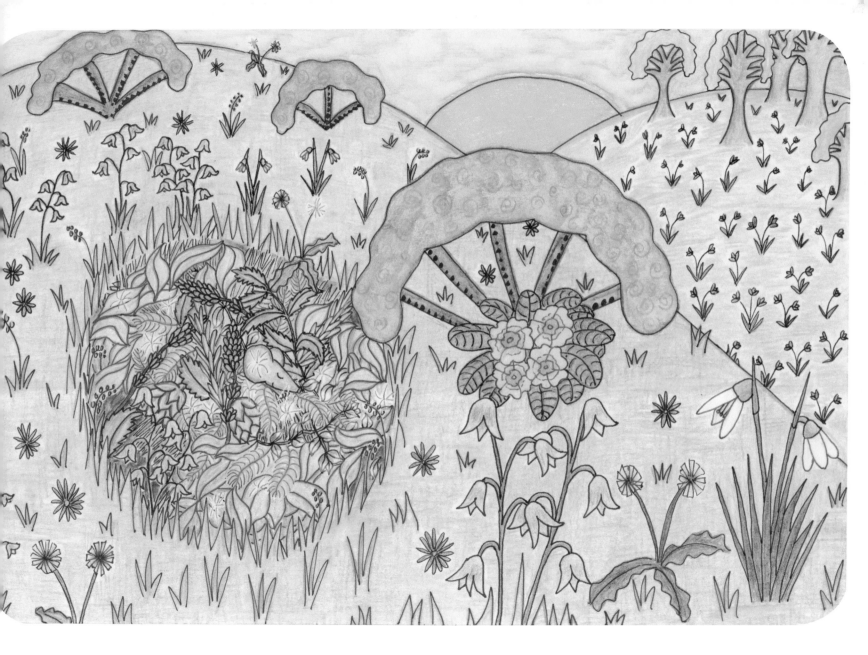